Health Benefits of Quinoa
For Cooking and Healing

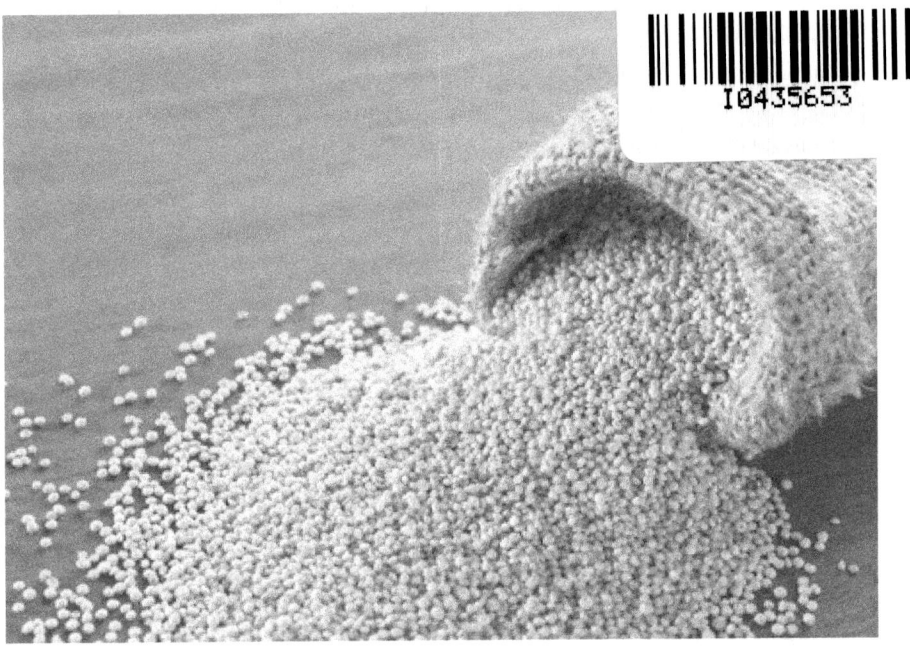

Health Learning Series
M. Usman
Mendon Cottage Books

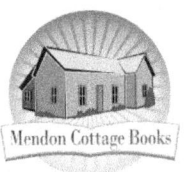

JD-Biz Publishing

Our books are available at

1. Amazon.com

2. Barnes and Noble

3. Itunes

4. Kobo

5. Smashwords

6. Google Play Books

Table of Contents

The Gold of the Incas

It was well over 5000 years ago when, high in the Andes Mountains, the Incas discovered and subsequently started to cultivate the warrior grain now known as Quinoa. Quinoa was extensively used in Incan culture and was known as the warrior grain by the indigenous people due to its stamina and power boosting properties. The performance enhancing secrets of Quinoa were buried by the Spanish conquistadors when they arrived in South America and destroyed fields of quinoa in order to annihilate the Incans, but quinoa survived and continued to grow in the wild mountains of the Andes. It wasn't until the 1980s, that two Americans stumbled over this ancient, super-nutritious food and began its cultivation in Colorado. Soon its popularity erupted and now quinoa is the subject of many food researchers along with natural medical practitioners. Its rejuvenating properties have been acknowledged by many and now are being used as much as possible. Apart from being refreshing, quinoa has shown the potential of being the curer of high-magnitude diseases like cancers, infections and neurological disorders.

Just keep on reading and uncover this mystery food and its amazing benefits.

Getting Started
Chapter 1: Intro

Quinoa is one of the oldest grains known to man. It is right up there with the likes of barley, faro and amaranth, but unlike most of the elderly grains it is exponentially gaining popularity among the general public. Pronounced as keen-wah, quinoa is actually a pseudocereal rather than a complete cereal, meaning that it is not entirely a member of the "grass family", but is also related to species like spinach, beetroot and tumbleweeds. However, pseudocereals can be treated just like other grains and can be milled and ground.

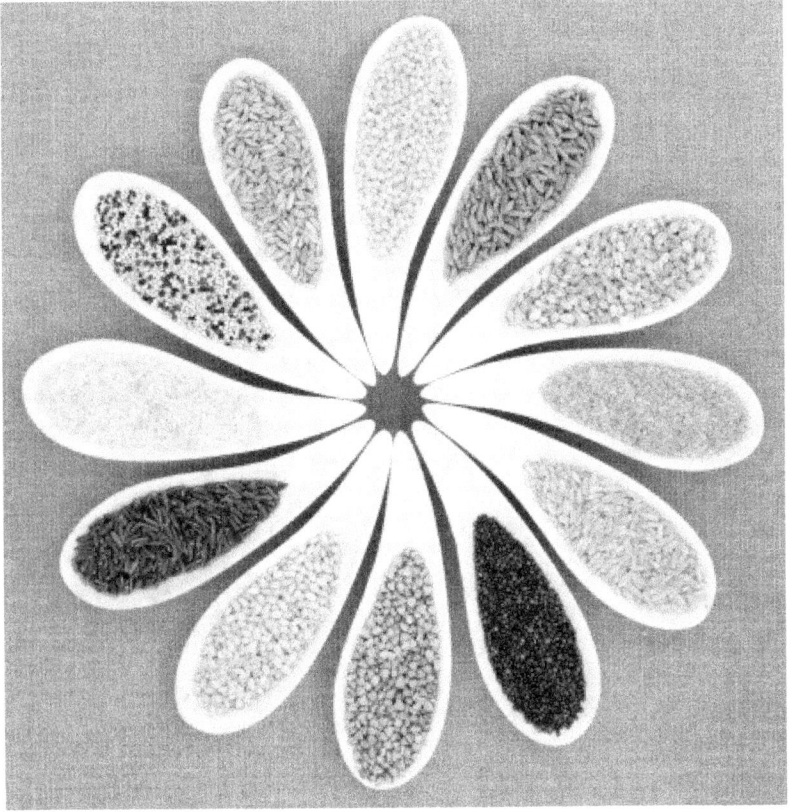

Quinoa is a tough crop and can easily thrive in poor conditions like sandy soil and extreme weather; however the preferred conditions for the crop are well-drained soil, neutral pH and mountainous regions. The plant itself reaches about 3-6 feet high and each plant produces almost a cup of seeds. All parts of the plant are edible, but the seeds are the most consumed ones. The seeds appear just like amaranth, are round in shape, smaller than millet seeds, and come in a rainbow of colors like red, purple, yellow and green. The most commonly available varieties of quinoa include red, black and white. Scientists have found renewed interest in quinoa due to a number of reasons, but the most intriguing one is its resistance and thriving nature in bad conditions. Along with its protein, fat and mineral content, quinoa can easily be chosen as a food in doomsday scenarios.

The following are the briefly described health benefits of the pseudocereal:

- Good for Diabetics – It is a well-known fact that a diabetic's condition is directly linked to the level of glucose in his/her body; as that level goes up, his/her condition worsens. Quinoa contains complex carbohydrates, which as the name suggest, are much harder for the body to break therefore, keeping the level of glucose almost constant. This keeps a diabetic satisfied in terms of food consumption and safe from any unwelcome condition.

- Maintains Cardiovascular functions – The researchers at University of Maryland have found that nutrients like Magnesium inside quinoa prove to be beneficial for the whole cardiovascular system by alleviating symptoms that result in heart diseases like hypertension and strokes.

- Works against migraines – Migraines can really cripple a person's life and take every bit of enjoyment out of the person. Phytonutrients in quinoa can help with this and lower the intensity of migraine attacks.

- No gluten – An increasing amount of people nowadays suffer from Celiac disease or gluten intolerance. Almost every grain contains gluten which makes it very hard for sufferers of celiac disease to deal with this problem. Fortunately, quinoa has no gluten and a lot of gluten intolerant people are terming it as "the best thing that could ever happen to them".

- Improves Digestion – Fiber is an essential part of the digestive system without which the whole body would become clogged, if you know what I mean! Like other grains, quinoa also contains a significant amount of fiber that makes it easier to digest food in a natural manner.

- Keeps you high on goodness – By eating junk food you really take the life out of a healthy body and make it slow, rusty and inactive. Quinoa is blessed with the right type of fats, proteins, carbohydrates and all the nutrients required for keeping the body in top notch shape; you will feel a marked difference upon regular consumption of this grain.

Chapter 2: Nutritional Worth

Quinoa, like many other grains, provides essential minerals, vitamins and fiber to the body which help in the maintenance of many of the body's systems. Quinoa, being a whole grain, provides the body with fiber that keeps it satisfied along with complex carbohydrates which are much higher in their nutritional worth than simple ones. Being dual in nature, quinoa's calorie content per 100 grams, i.e. 368 calories are similar to many major cereals like maize, rice and wheat and pulses like mung bean, chickpea and cowpea. It is filled with the extremely beneficial protein lysine which is essential for tissue growth in the body; 100 grams of quinoa packs about 14-18 grams of proteins.

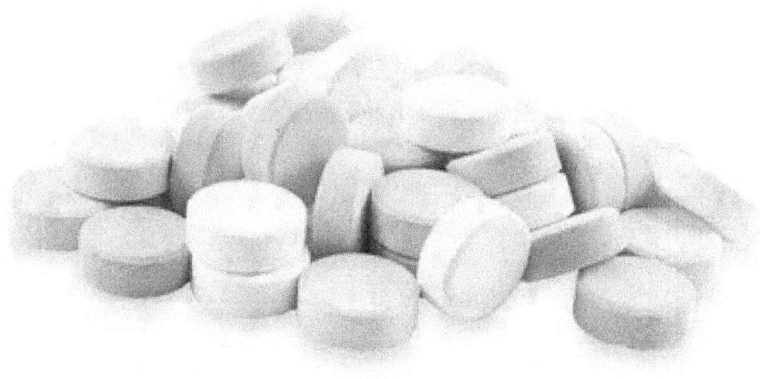

Quinoa is a great source of both soluble and insoluble fiber that has several benefits, notably to the digestive system. Dietary fiber increases the bulkiness of quinoa and improves the digestive system by increasing the rate of movement through the gut. That's not the only benefit of fiber; as fiber also prevents colorectal cancer by binding to hazardous toxins as soon as they are excreted in the gut. It also binds to chemicals that result in lesser production of LDL cholesterol.

Quinoa does a good job at providing the body with B-vitamins, vitamin E and essential fatty acids as well. About 25% of quinoa's fatty acid comes from oleic acid which is a heart healthy fat that improves the cardiovascular position of the body. The leaves of quinoa are great sources of vitamin A, folates and antioxidants like carotene, Zeaxanthin, etc.; the latter are absolutely necessary for the body as without them, the body won't be able to thrive against infections, aging and neurological diseases.

Lastly, quinoa contains a wide array of minerals like copper, calcium, iron, manganese, potassium and magnesium that are all required by the body in one place or another.

i. Copper is required in the production of red blood cells while iron is required in their formation.

ii. Magnesium relaxes the blood vessels going to the brain and works against depression.

iii. Zinc is a helping substance in compounds that regulate the enhancement of cells and nucleic acid syntheses.

iv. Potassium controls the body fluids that in turn control the heart rate.

v. Manganese is used by the body as an antioxidant.

A detailed account of the nutritional wellness of **uncooked quinoa** is given in the following table. The amount taken is that of a single cup or 170 grams.

Calorie Information		
Nutrient	**Amount**	**% DV**
Total Calories	626 (2621 kJ)	31%
From Carbohydrates	437 (1830 kJ)	
From Fat	92.9 (389 kJ)	
From Proteins	96.0 (402 kJ)	
Carbohydrates		
Nutrient	**Amount**	**% DV**
Total Carbohydrates	109 g	36%

Dietary Fiber	11.9 g	48%
Starch	88.8 g	
Sugar	~	

Fats & Fatty Acids

Nutrient	Amount	% DV
Total Fat	10.3 g	16%
Saturated Fat	1.2 g	6%
Mono-saturated Fat	2.7 g	
Polyunsaturated Fat	5.6 g	
Total Omega-3 Fatty acids	522 mg	
Total Omega-6 Fatty acids	5061 mg	

Proteins

Nutrient	Amount	% DV
Protein	24.0 g	48%

Vitamins

Nutrient	Amount	% DV
Vitamin A	23.8 IU	0%
Vitamin C	~	~
Vitamin E	4.1 mg	21%
Vitamin K	0.0 mcg	0%
Thiamin	0.6 mg	41%
Riboflavin	0.5 mg	32%
Niacin	2.6 mg	13%
Vitamin B6	0.8 mg	41%
Folate	313 mcg	78%
Vitamin B12	0.0 mg	0%
Pantothenic Acid	1.3 mg	13%
Choline	119 mg	
Betaine	1072 mg	

Minerals

Nutrient	Amount	% DV
Calcium	79.9 mg	8%
Iron	7.8 mg	43%
Magnesium	335 mg	84%
Phosphorus	777 mg	78%
Potassium	957 mg	27%
Sodium	8.5 mg	0%

Zinc	5.3 mg	35%
Copper	1.0 mg	50%
Manganese	3.5 mg	173%
Selenium	14.4 mcg	21%

The following is a table stating the nutritional worth of 1 cup of **cooked quinoa** worth 185 grams:

Calorie Information		
Nutrient	**Amount**	**% DV**
Total Calories	222 (929 kJ)	2%
From Carbohydrates	157 (657 kJ)	
From Fat	32.0 (134 kJ)	
From Proteins	32.6 (136 kJ)	
Carbohydrates		
Nutrient	**Amount**	**% DV**
Total Carbohydrates	39.4 g	13%
Dietary Fiber	5.2 g	21%
Starch	32.6 g	
Sugar	~	
Fats & Fatty Acids		
Nutrient	**Amount**	**% DV**
Total Fat	3.6 g	5%
Saturated Fat	~	~
Mono-saturated Fat	~	
Polyunsaturated Fat	~	
Total Omega-3 Fatty acids	~	
Total Omega-6 Fatty acids	~	
Proteins		
Nutrient	**Amount**	**% DV**
Protein	8.1 g	16%
Vitamins		
Nutrient	**Amount**	**% DV**
Vitamin A	9.3 IU	0%
Vitamin C	0.0 mg	0%
Vitamin E	1.2 mg	6%

Vitamin K	~	~
Thiamin	0.2 mg	13%
Riboflavin	0.2 mg	12%
Niacin	0.8 mg	5%
Vitamin B6	0.2 mg	12%
Folate	77.7 mcg	19%
Vitamin B12	0.0 mg	0%
Pantothenic Acid	~	~
Choline	~	
Betaine	~	
Minerals		
Nutrient	**Amount**	**% DV**
Calcium	31.5 mg	3%
Iron	2.8 mg	15%
Magnesium	118 mg	30%
Phosphorus	281 mg	28%
Potassium	318 mg	9%
Sodium	13.0 mg	1%
Zinc	2.0 mg	13%
Copper	0.4 mg	18%
Manganese	1.2 mg	58%
Selenium	5.2 mcg	7%

It can be clearly seen that cooking quinoa, diminishes it of its fatty acids, both omega-3 and omega-6, therefore, if you are looking for fatty acids, uncooked quinoa will serve you best.

Chapter 3: Selection & Storage

Before going in to the details of the selection process, one must know about the types of quinoa:

i.   White quinoa:

This is the most common type of quinoa available in the market and is commonly referred to as just 'quinoa'. It has a white color that distinctly separates it from other grains.

ii.   Red quinoa:

As the name suggests, it is red in color and holds its shape after cooking making it more suitable for recipes that involve cooking where the shape is necessary.

iii.   Black quinoa:

This one is a bit sweeter and earthier with a striking black color after it has been cooked.

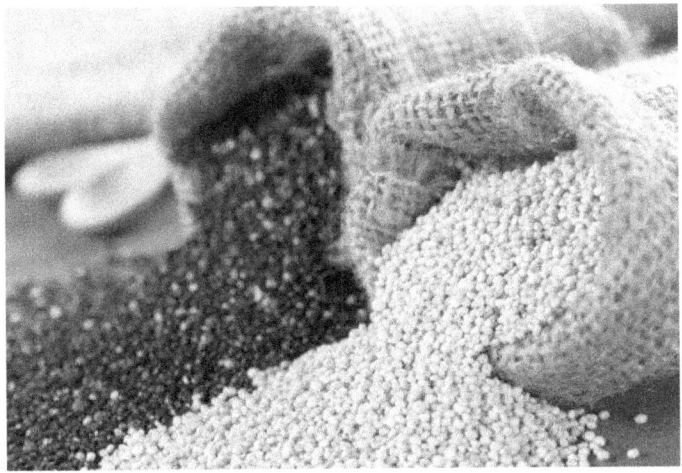

All types of quinoa are generally available in either prepackaged containers or bulk bins. When purchasing from bins, make sure that the bins are properly covered and kept in a dry place; moreover, the store should have a high turnover rate as this would guarantee freshness. When deciding about the quantity to purchase, remember that quinoa expands to several time its original size. Either way, look for fine, dry grains that are similar in size to millets. At home, store the grains in an air-tight container in a cool place where they will easily remain fresh for several months. Ground quinoa should be stored in an air-tight container, as well, as it can rapidly oxidize after coming in contact with air. Quinoa can also be stored in a refrigerator where it will keep for 3-6 months without going rancid.

Health Benefits

Chapter 1: Cholesterol

Cholesterol is both our friend and our enemy – at optimum levels it is absolutely necessary for the body, but if it gets too high, it can become a big problem, especially for the heart. Cholesterol is found in every cell and has four main functions:

i.   Constitutes the structure of the cell wall.

ii.   Produces digestive acids in the gut.

iii.   Allows the production of vitamin D.

iv.   Allows the production of specific hormones in the body.

There are two basic types of cholesterol, which will decide the basis of this chapter:

    i.   Low density lipoprotein cholesterol or LDL cholesterol which is also known as bad cholesterol.

    ii.   High density lipoprotein cholesterol or HDL cholesterol which is known as good cholesterol.

LDL cholesterol is the type of cholesterol which causes heavy damage to the body and therefore, should be handled with caution. High levels of LDL cholesterol can lead to cardiovascular risks including heart attack, stroke and hypertension. Quinoa comes in to save the day with its right quantity and quality fiber content which is essential for the maintenance of optimum health. When fiber from quinoa is consumed, it combines with the liver's bile acids to produce a jelly-like product during bowel movements. The liver requires stored cholesterol to produce more bile acids. Therefore, these stores are depleted by the help of fiber's binding to bile acids. The body's total cholesterol, as well as, bad cholesterol level drops proving quinoa to be a healthy food. In particular, quinoa contains very little cholesterol making it a great alternative to fat rich foods like lean meat and proteins that increase the LDL cholesterol levels in the body leading to problems like heart failure, coronary heart disease and heart attacks. Coronary heart disease starts up with the buildup of excess cholesterol and fat in the blood which blocks the inner walls of the blood vessels, resulting in a decrease in the rate of oxygen transfer throughout the body. The arteries become narrower each day and a condition known as atherosclerosis starts to develop. When the body gets quinoa, the LDL cholesterol is dealt with and the arteries return back to their normal function; this conclusively deals with the risk of cardiovascular diseases.

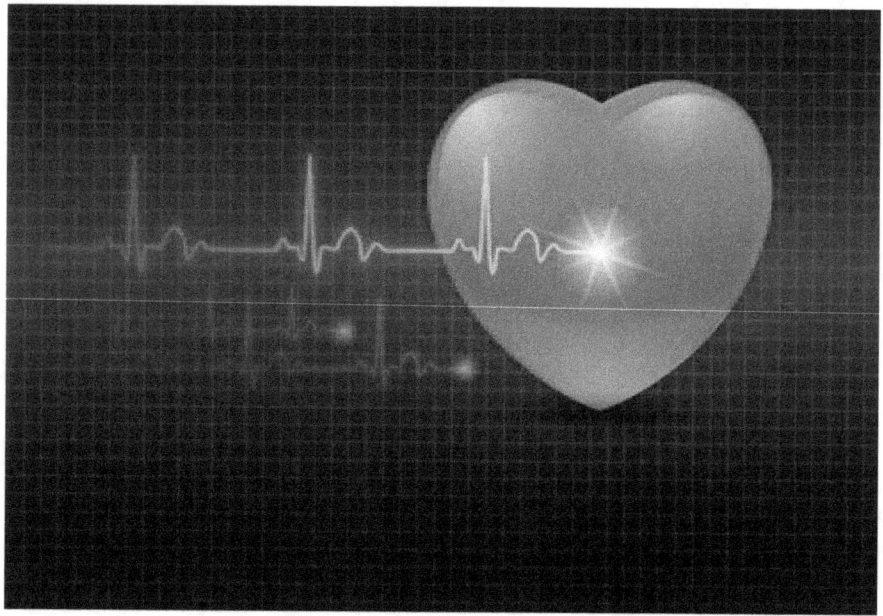

Human trials are still underway but a 2010 study conducted in the Netherlands analyzed the lipid profile, protein metabolism, and glucose levels in rats fed with quinoa. The final analysis of the blood of each rat indicated that the seeds reduced the levels of total cholesterol by 26% compared to the neutral group, along with 11% reduction in triglycerides. Also, when quinoa seeds were added to the diet of the rats, the loss of HDL cholesterol also decreased showing that quinoa provided the body with 2 benefits at the same time by making sure that nothing good gets taken out of the body.

Chapter 2: Migraines

A migraine is a severely painful headache that is accompanied by warning signs like blind spots, flashes of light, tingling in the limbs, vomiting and nausea. A migraine is characterized by excruciating pain that may last for hours or days. An episode of migraine takes place from a combination of events that include the enlargement of blood vessels along with the release of chemicals from nerve fibers that wind around these vessels. The artery that enlarges is located just outside the skull, under the skin of the temple which becomes the epicenter of the whole episode.

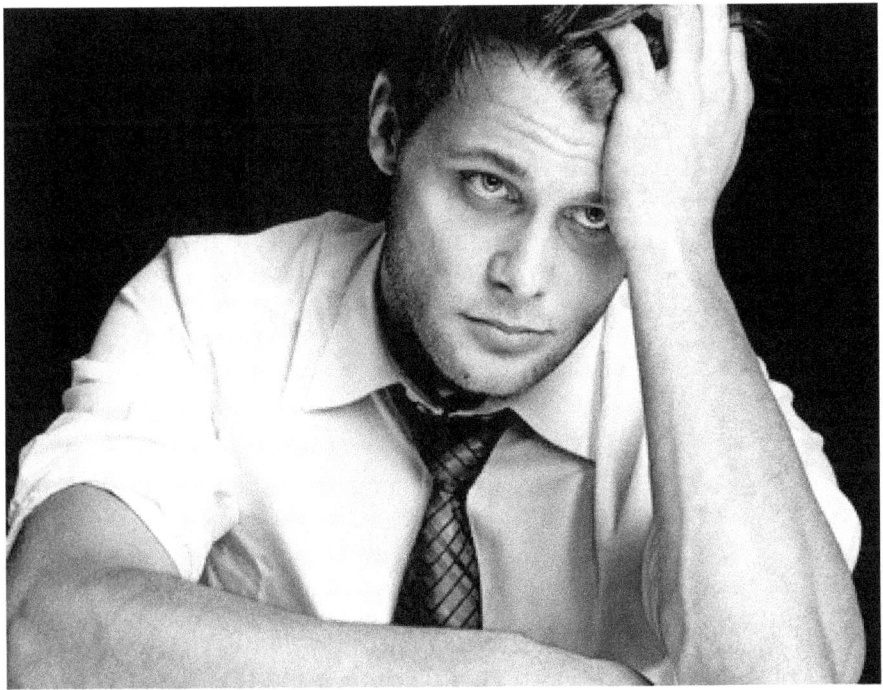

Quinoa may not be the first food that comes to one's mind when talking about migraine, but people who have used this as a solution will tell you that it is very effective. Migraines are relieved by two nutrients, namely, riboflavin and magnesium, both of which are abundantly found in quinoa. Magnesium is well known for its ability to aid in the reduction of headaches by reducing the rigidness of blood vessels, making them more toned and flexible. To increase its amount in the body, an adequate amount of riboflavin or vitamin B6 is required. Moreover, another cause of migraine is thought to be constipation; therefore, quinoa seems to be the right choice as it is very robust in dealing with digestive issues!

A study conducted in the 2010 issue of the Journal of Pain Research showed that quinoa indeed helped in alleviating migraine pain. The study was designed to evaluate the different dietary factors that affect the frequency and intensity of pain felt by migraine patients. Fifty consecutive Turkish patients who consisted of 13 men and 37 women were first diagnosed with migraines and then randomly divided into two groups. The first group was treated with riboflavin, metoprolol and naproxen sodium, just at the start and the end of the attacks. The second group was supplied with a comprehensive list of items along with the same medical protocol as the first group. At the end of the study it was found that riboflavin effectively reduced pain in patients of migraines; also the second group resorted to much less use of medical equipment due to effectiveness of vitamin B2. It was concluded that foods rich in vitamin B2 have the ability to decrease the duration, intensity and frequency of migraine attacks.

Chapter 3: Weight Loss

Quinoa is really having a moment right now. Along with curing high magnitude diseases, it is now being found out that quinoa helps with weight loss. The reason behind this discovery is simple: quinoa is quite rich in complex carbohydrates plus complete proteins. Fiona Hunter, an expert nutritionist, has stated that Quinoa has a low glycemic index and has twice as much protein as rice, making it a great diet for people who want to lose fat but keep their protein. The logic behind quinoa's weight losing benefit can be divided into four parts:

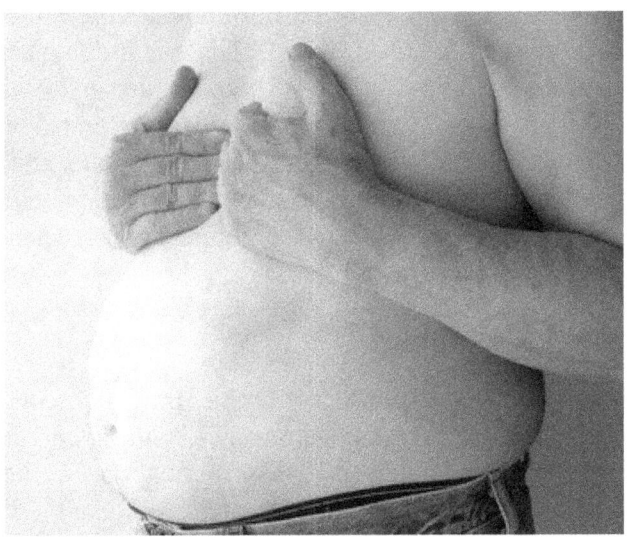

i. **Vitamins:**

Quinoa is rich in eight essential amino acids, vitamins, and minerals like magnesium, iron and calcium. Iron and vitamin B12 have a synergistic effect, which is efficient energy production that leads to weight loss. A low presence of B vitamins in the body bogs down the loss of extra weight as synthesis of nutrients become very inefficient. Furthermore, the minerals and vitamins ensure a steady stream of energy which results in buildup of all parts of the body including the bones and teeth and not just muscles.

ii. **Satiating:**

As quinoa is rich in the right fiber and proteins, it can make you feel much fuller than unhealthy foods that include both processed-natural and over-processed junk foods. Quinoa contains almost seven grams of proteins in a single serving and six grams of fiber that is helpful for everyone, especially vegetarians, who are trying to lose weight but have trouble filling them up. Dietary fiber found in quinoa binds to fat as well as cholesterol making it less likely for the fat to become a part of the body. This is one mechanism by which quinoa acts on the body.

iii.   Low Glycemic Index:

As stated above, quinoa has a low GI. GI indicates the effect of carbohydrates on blood glucose. A low glycemic index means that the food won't spike your blood sugar. When the glucose level in your blood rises, it causes you to crave for more carbohydrates or sugar. When the sugar levels are unbalanced, staying on a diet and following it becomes extremely difficult due to increased frequency of these cravings. Quinoa ranks 35 on the glycemic index, and when compared to other food, is quite low.

iv.   Low Calorie:

Quinoa is also low in calories as stated in the previous section. One serving of cooked quinoa contains almost 172 calories. Even if you consumed two or three whole servings of quinoa, you would still be eating less, in terms of calories, than a plate of pasta. You don't have to worry about overeating quinoa, but still you must consider it (explained later). For a great low quality meal, combine quinoa with a salad and beans.

Although eating quinoa can shed off extra pounds from your body, eating too much will cause a hindrance in weight loss. For instance, 4 cups of quinoa would provide you with 888 calories which would be more than half of the daily requirement when following a 1200 – 1600 calorie weight loss plan. Remember moderation is always the key to eating foods. The amount of quinoa you eat should be dependent on your weight loss plan. The 2010 Dietary Guidelines for Americans advises you to eat 4 ounces of the grain on a daily basis in the case of a 1200 calorie diet plan and subsequently 5 ounces if following a 1400 – 1600 calorie plan. An ounce equivalent of the grain equals ½ cup quinoa or 1 cup breakfast cereal.

Chapter # 4: Colorectal Cancer

Cancer is a disease, or more precisely a name, for a group of diseases that affect the body by uncontrolled growth of abnormal cells. Many cancers start out as simple harmless tumors that turn bad and spread throughout the body. Tumors grow and interfere with normal functions like nervous, digestive and circulatory systems that release hormones, altering major body functions. A tumor becomes real danger for the body when:

> i.   A cancerous cell manages to escape its confinement and move in the body using the lymph system, destroying healthy tissues.

ii.   A cancerous cell manages to divide and grow.

There are over 100 different types of cancer that are named after the organ they affect. One such cancer is colon cancer. This is caused and affected by a number of factors with chronic inflammation topping the list. Chronic inflammation is caused by a high level of toxins in the food, nutritional deficiency, or even both. The key to reducing chances of colon cancer is by eliminating foods that cause agitation and inflammation in the first place. After that you can start consuming foods that are anti-inflammatory in nature and can repair the damage caused by the underlying toxins. Quinoa is a food that has abundant amounts of high quality anti-inflammatories; these are known as saponins. Saponins are bitter tasting, water soluble compounds found in the outer part of the seed coat layer of the grain. The saponins have showed both antioxidant and anti-inflammatory behavior, but it is worth nothing that soaking, boiling and milling will reduce their presence in general. In general, the relationship between anti-inflammatory benefits of quinoa and saponins levels is still be clarified, however the anti-inflammatory properties of quinoa are a sure thing.

Another mechanism by which quinoa acts is by using the power of its dietary fiber. The fiber offered by quinoa is insoluble, meaning it can't dissolve in water. This particular type of fiber regulates bowel movements by passing through one's intestinal tract and helping the stool move more viscously through the colon. This waste contains carcinogens which are compounds that affect the intestinal cells. In addition, a bacterium tends to break down fiber, as a result of which a chemical that inhibits cancer growth is produced.

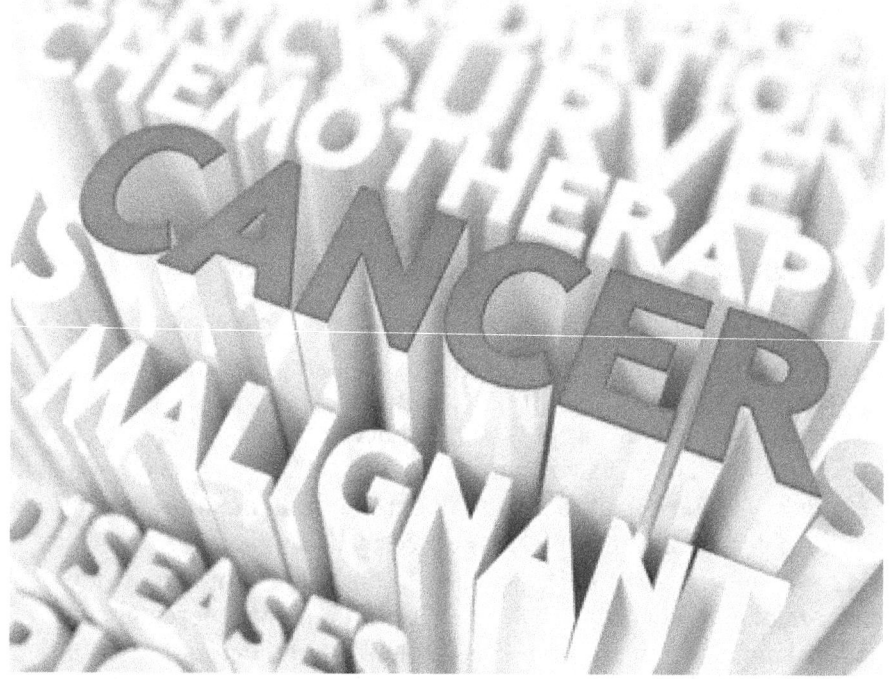

The U.S. Polyp Prevention trial carried out from 1991 – 1998 examined the effect of a low fat, high fiber diet in almost 2000 participants. This study was published in the American Journal of Epidemiology and showed a wide range of variation in the level of effectiveness of fiber. Researchers recorded a 35% percent reduced recurrence of colorectal cancer compared to control groups. Insoluble fiber also works against cancers like breast, mouth and throat but researches on these particular cancers is still underway.

Recipes
Chapter 1: Blueberry Lemon Breakfast Quinoa
Makes: 2 servings

Prep time: 5 minutes

Cooking time: 25 minutes

Ingredients:

- 1 cup quinoa

- 2 cups non-fat milk

- ½ lemon

- 1 pinch salt

- 2 teaspoons flax seed

- 3 tablespoons maple syrup

Directions:

First, rinse quinoa in a strainer with some cold water in order to remove its bitterness; do this until there is no froth. Then, heat the milk in a saucepan over medium intensity heat until it turns warm, which will take about 3 minutes. Stir in the quinoa and salt into the milk and simmer for about 20 minutes or until much of the liquid is absorbed. Remove the saucepan from heat, stir in the maple syrup, lemon zest plus quinoa and fold the blueberries into the mixture. Finally, divide the quinoa mixture in 2 bowls and top each one with a teaspoon of flax; serve.

Chapter # 2: Quinoa Tabbouleh

Makes: 4 servings

Prep time: 15 minutes

Cooking time: 15 minutes

Ingredients:

- 2 cups water
- 3 diced tomatoes
- 1 cup quinoa
- 1 diced cucumber
- 1 pinch salt
- 2 diced bunches green onions
- ¼ cup olive oil
- 2 grated carrots
- ½ teaspoon salt
- 1 cup chopped parsley
- ¼ cup lemon juice

Directions:

In a saucepan, boil the water and add quinoa and a pinch of salt. Reduce heat to low and simmer for 15 minutes. Allow the saucepan to cool to room temperature while fluffing with a fork. Meanwhile, combine olive oil, lemon juice, sea salt, tomatoes, green onions, cucumber, parsley and carrots in a large bowl and stir in the cooled quinoa.

Chapter # 3: Turkey & Quinoa Meatloaf

Makes: 5 servings

Prep time: 30 minutes

Cooking time: 50 minutes

Ingredients:

- ¼ cup quinoa
- 2 tablespoons Worcestershire sauce
- ½ cup water
- 1 egg
- 1 teaspoon olive oil
- 1 ½ teaspoons salt
- 1 small onion
- 1 teaspoon ground black pepper
- 1 large clove
- 2 tablespoons brown sugar
- 1 package ground turkey, 20 ounce
- 2 teaspoons Worcestershire sauce
- 1 tablespoon tomato sauce
- 1 tablespoon hot pepper sauce
- 1 teaspoon water

Directions:

Bring the water and quinoa to a boil in a saucepan and reduce the heat to medium after boiling starts; cover and simmer until the quinoa turns tender and all the water has been absorbed. Set aside so it can cool down. Preheat an oven to 175 degrees Celsius and start heating the olive oil in a skillet. Stir in the onion and cook it until it softens and turns translucent. Add the garlic and remove from heat after one minute. Stir the turkey, cooked quinoa, tomato paste, onions, 2 tablespoons Worcestershire, egg, hot sauce, salt and pepper in a large bowl and shape it into a loaf on foil. Combine the brown sugar, 1 teaspoon water with 2 teaspoons Worcestershire and rub the paste over the meatloaf. Bake the meatloaf until it is no longer pink which will take 50 minutes. Let the meatloaf cook for another 10 minutes before serving.

Chapter # 4: Chicken with Quinoa & Veggies

Makes: 4 servings

Prep time: 30 minutes

Cooking time: 25 minutes

Ingredients:

- 1 cup rinsed quinoa
- 2 tablespoons olive oil
- 2 cups chicken broth
- 1 diced zucchini
- 1 diced tomato
- 2 tablespoons olive oil
- 4 ounces crumbled cheese
- 2 garlic scapes
- 8 fresh basil leaves
- 1 small onion
- 1 tablespoon lime juice
- 2 skinless, boneless chicken

Directions:

Boil the chicken broth and quinoa in a saucepan; reduce the heat to simmer and cover the pan afterwards. Let it simmer until the quinoa turns fluffy, broth is absorbed, and white line is visible on the grain. Heat 2 tablespoons of olive oil and cook the garlic scapes plus onion in a skillet for 5 minutes. Stir in the chicken breasts and cook it until it turns pink in the middle which will take about 5 more minutes. Remove the chicken meat and pour 2 more tablespoons of olive oil in a skillet and cook the zucchini and tomato for 7 minutes. Place the chicken back in the skillet and sprinkle basil leaves, lime juice and feta cheese. Cook the chicken for 10 more minutes and serve with hot quinoa.

Chapter # 5: Quinoa Almond Pilaf

Makes: 3 servings

Prep time: 20 minutes

Cooking time: 25 minutes

Ingredients:

- ½ cup rinsed & drained quinoa

- 1 cup cold water

- 8 almonds, chopped

- 1 small tomato

- ¼ teaspoon salt

- 2 tablespoons raisins

- 1/8 teaspoon salt

- 3 tablespoons olive oil

- 1 celery rib

- 1/8 teaspoon black pepper

- 1 small chopped onion

- 1/8 teaspoon thyme

- 1 chopped carrot

- 1/8 teaspoon oregano

- 1 minced garlic clove

- 1/8 teaspoon dried oregano

- 1 pinch coarse salt

Directions:

Combine cold water, salt and quinoa in a saucepan and bring it to a boil; reduce the heat to medium low and place a cover on the saucepan afterwards. Cook until the liquid becomes fully absorbed, which will take about 15 minutes. Heat the olive oil over medium heat in a skillet and cook the onion, carrot, celery and garlic in hot olive oil until the onion turns translucent which will take 5 minutes. Stir in the tomato, almonds, raisins, pepper, thyme, salt and oregano into the mixture and cook for 1 more minute. Fluff the quinoa with a fork and stir it into the mixture; now cook the quinoa for 30 seconds. Finally, divide the mixture, evenly between 3 plates and sprinkle sea salt over each plate for a surprising crunch of saltiness!

Chapter # 6: Spanish Quinoa

Makes: 4 cups

Prep time: 20 minutes

Cooking time: 40 minutes

Ingredients:

- 2 tablespoons vegetable oil

- 1 can tomato sauce

- 1 cup uncooked quinoa

- 2 ½ cups of water

- 1 medium, finely chopped onions

- 1 teaspoon chili powder

- ¼ teaspoon garlic powder

- 3 minced garlic cloves

- ¼ teaspoon cumin

- 1 small green bell pepper

Directions:

Heat the vegetable oil in a saucepan over medium heat and stir in the quinoa, garlic, onion and green pepper; cook for 5 – 10 minutes until the onion is tender and then stir in tomato sauce along with water. Season with chili powder, cumin and garlic and bring it to a boil. Finally reduce the heat to low and simmer the mixture until the quinoa turns tender which will take 30 minutes. Stir in the quinoa in short intervals until it becomes fully cooked.

Conclusion

The 'Gold of the Incas' is the new super food and is being regarded highly by many researchers around the globe. The crop that once came close to extinction is now being cultivated more and more due to ever increasing popularity and newly discovered health benefits. Quinoa is being revered by researchers so much, because of its abundant, but more importantly, unique reservoir of nutrients. New benefits of the psuedograin are being discovered everyday against diseases that cost thousands to the general public or are incurable, i.e. cancer, heart disease, etc. Everything has been made available to you and it's up to you now to stay motivated and change your lifestyle and reap the benefits of this food that gives you the best of both worlds.

And if nothing suits you, just eat it for its culinary blessedness!

Author Bio

Muhammad Usman is a distinguished medical graduate of Allama Iqbal medical college (AIMC). He is a professional writer who has been in the field for more than 4 years. During this time he has produced 10,000+ articles, blogs and eBooks on various niches related to diseases, health, fitness, nutrition and well-being. He is a regular contributor to several journals related to medicine and surgery. He is the editor of several journals and newspapers.

Check out some of the other JD-Biz Publishing books
Gardening Series on Amazon

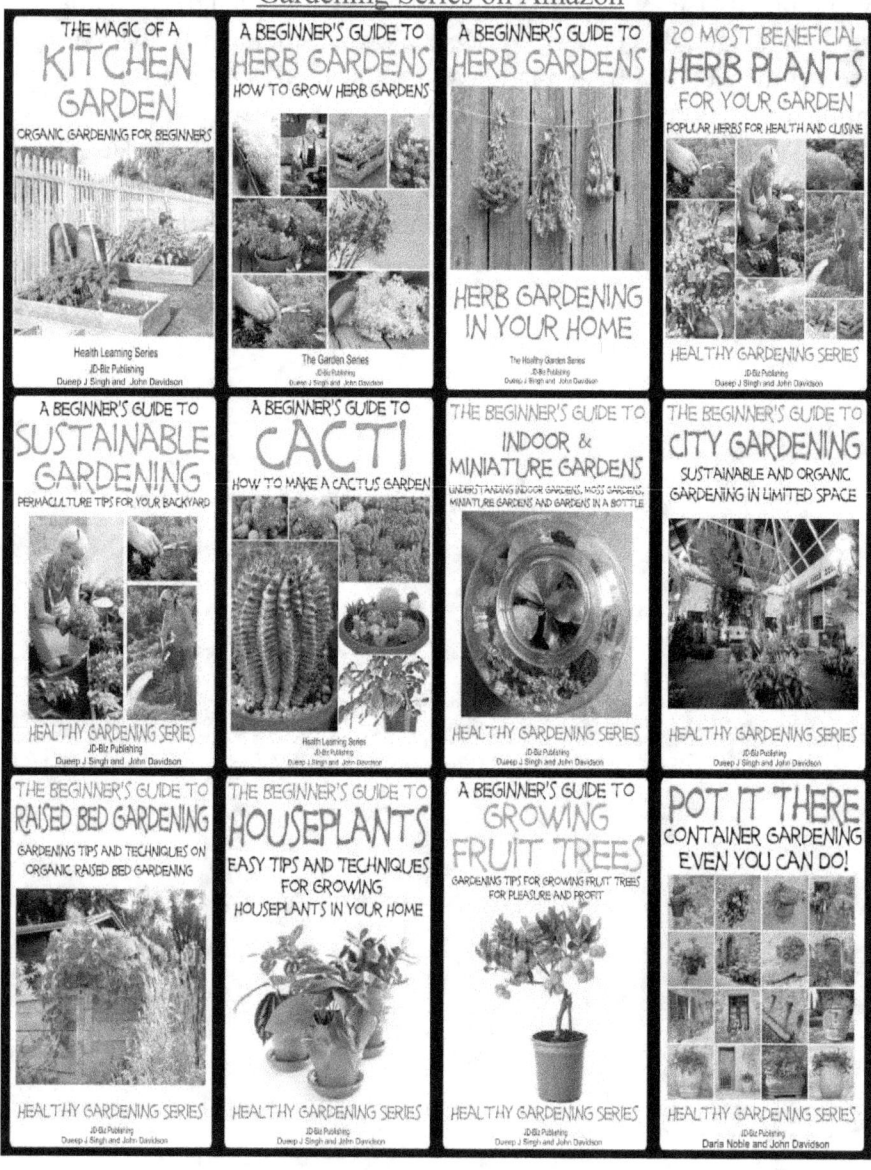

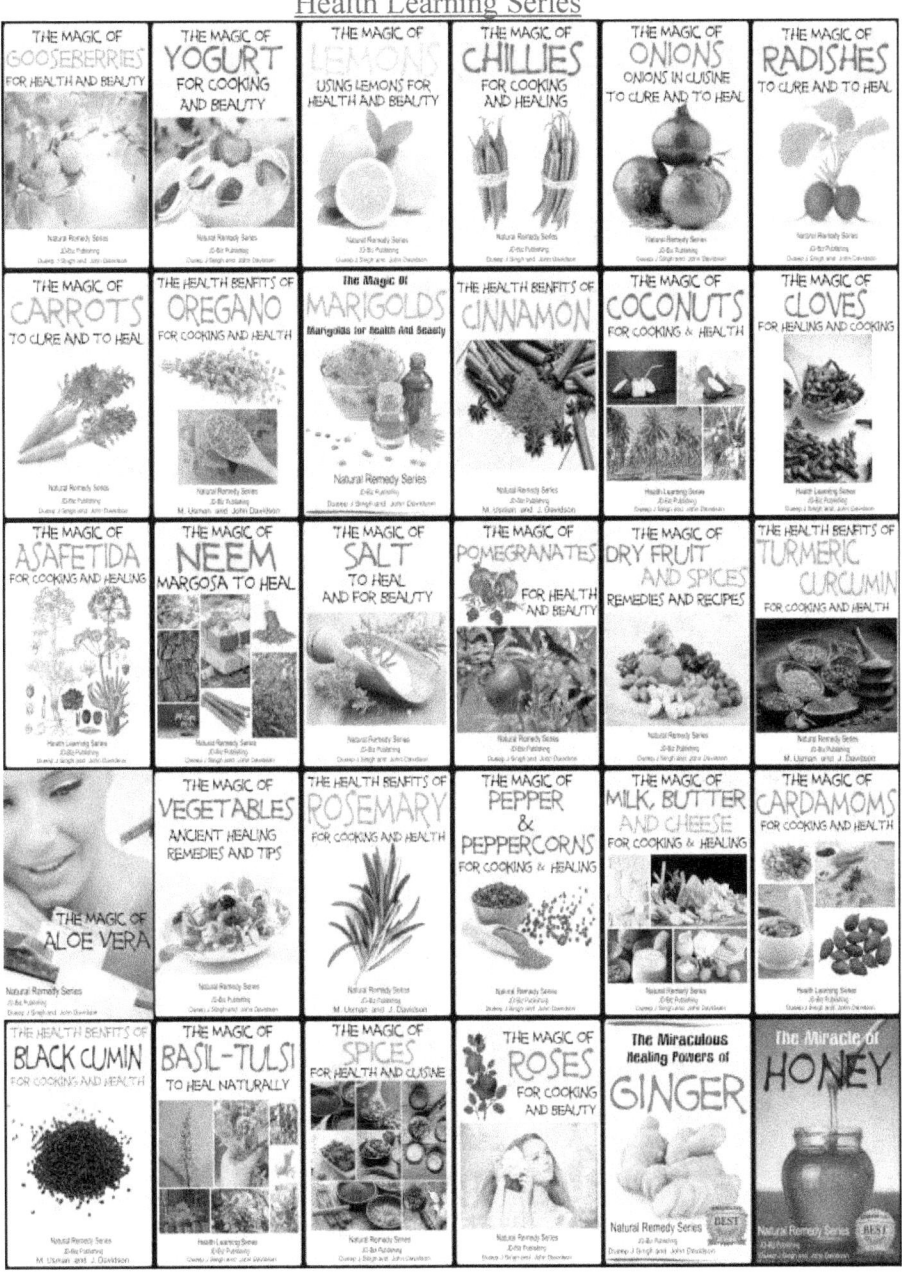

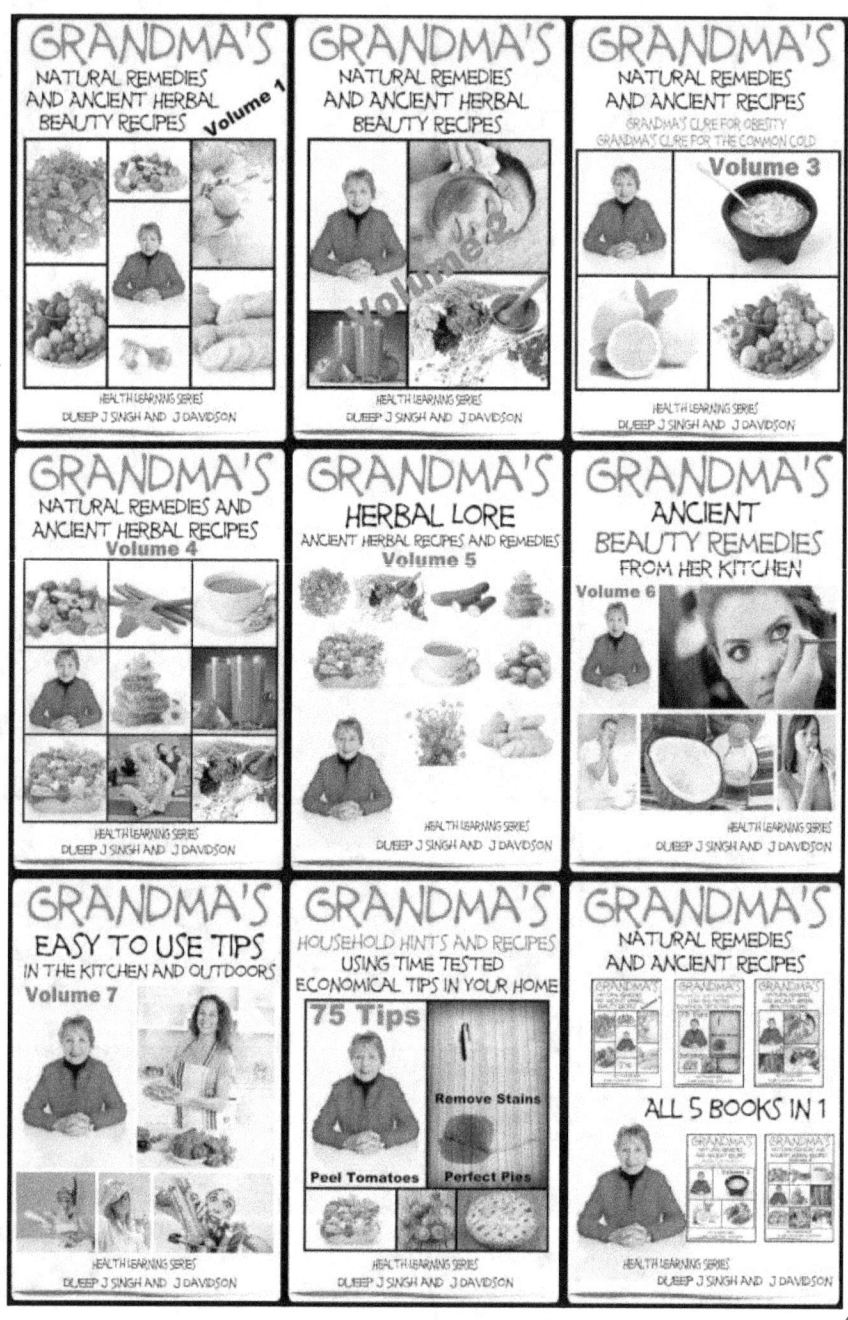

Co untry Life Books

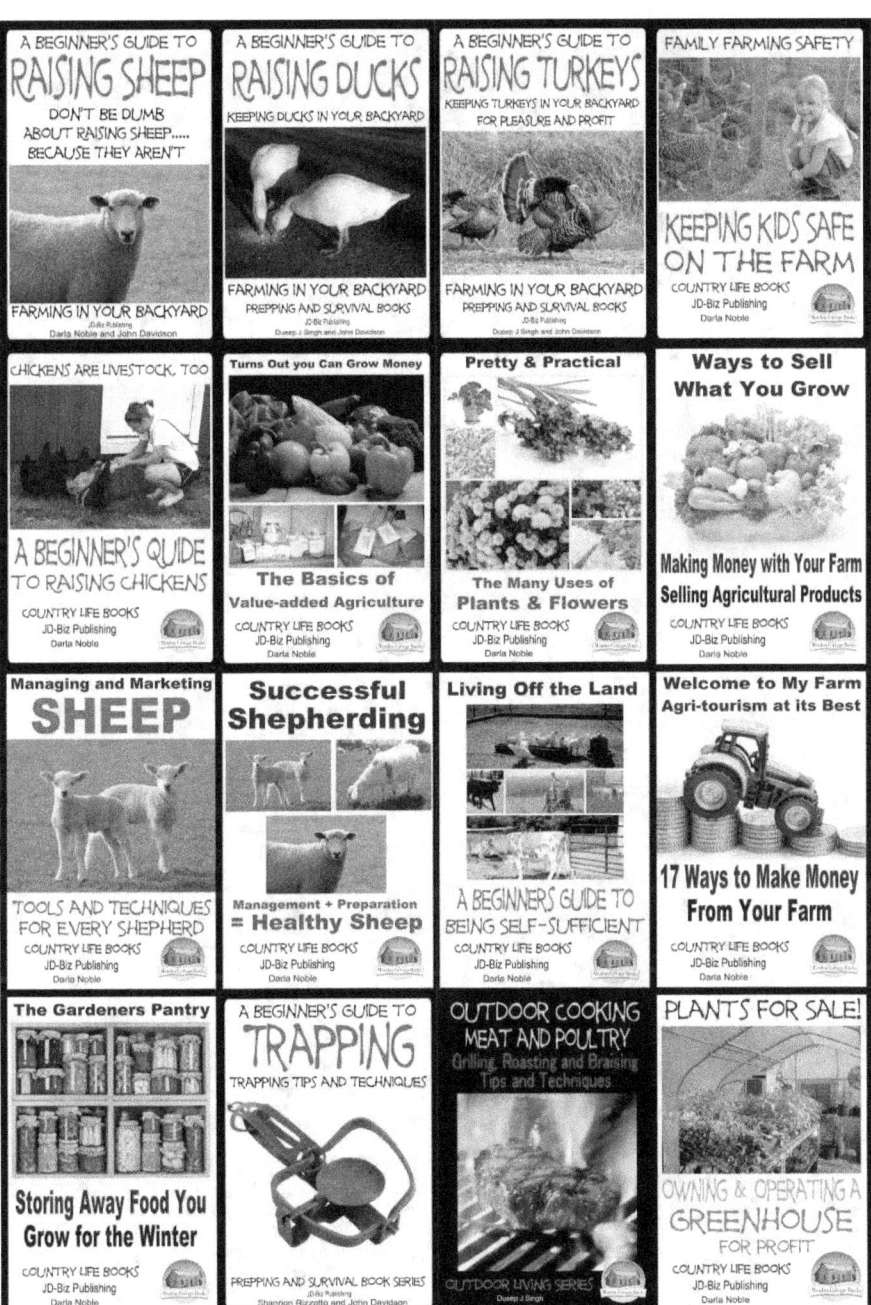

Health Learning Series

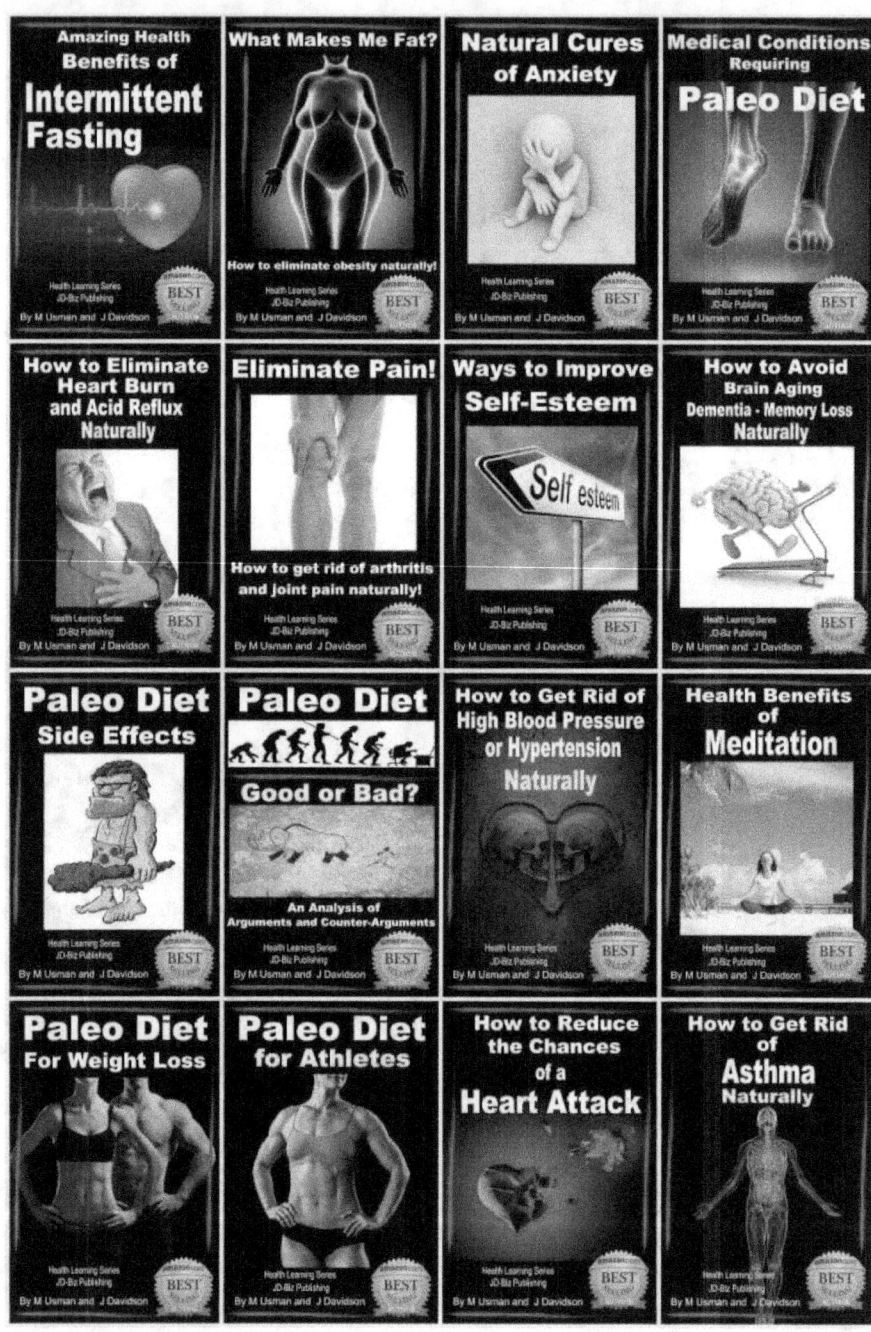

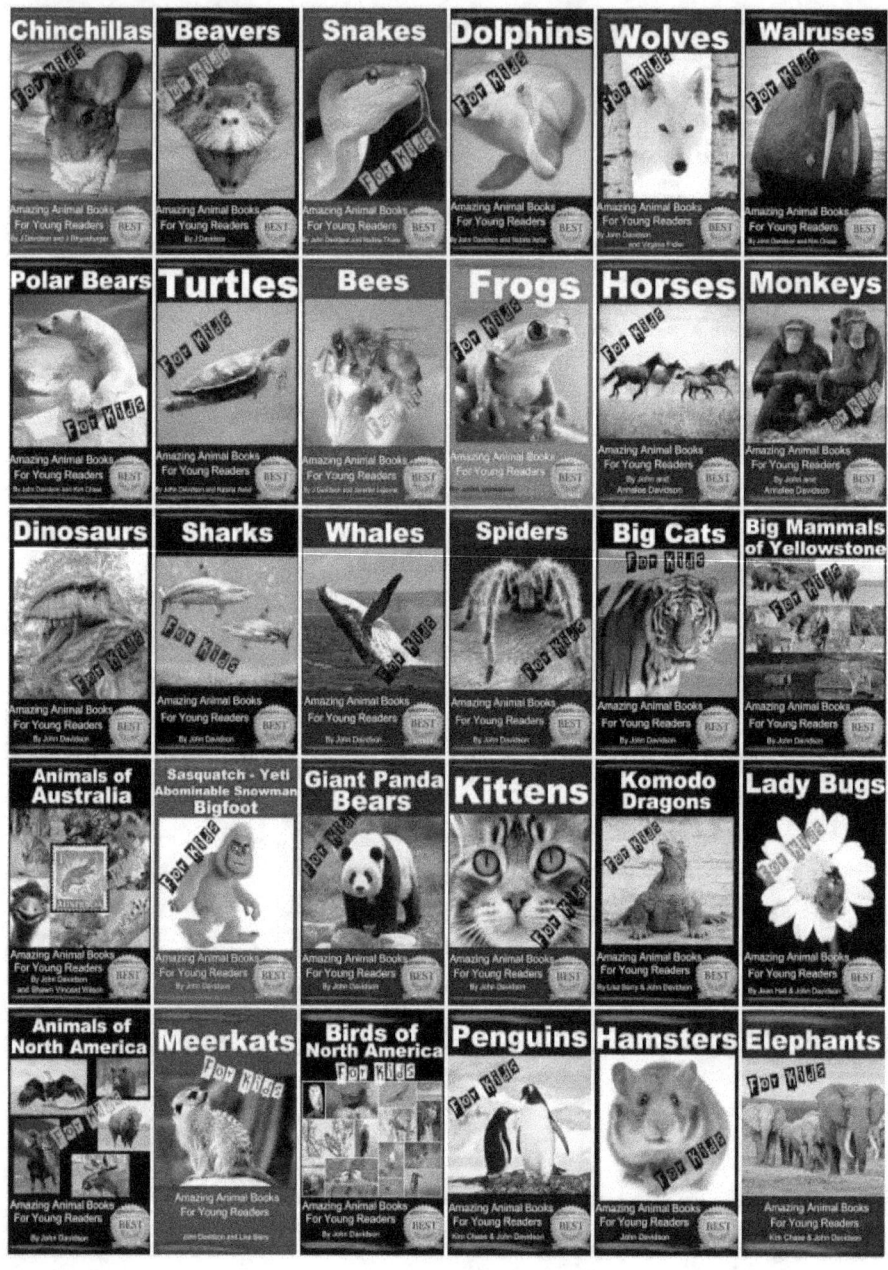

Learn To Draw Series

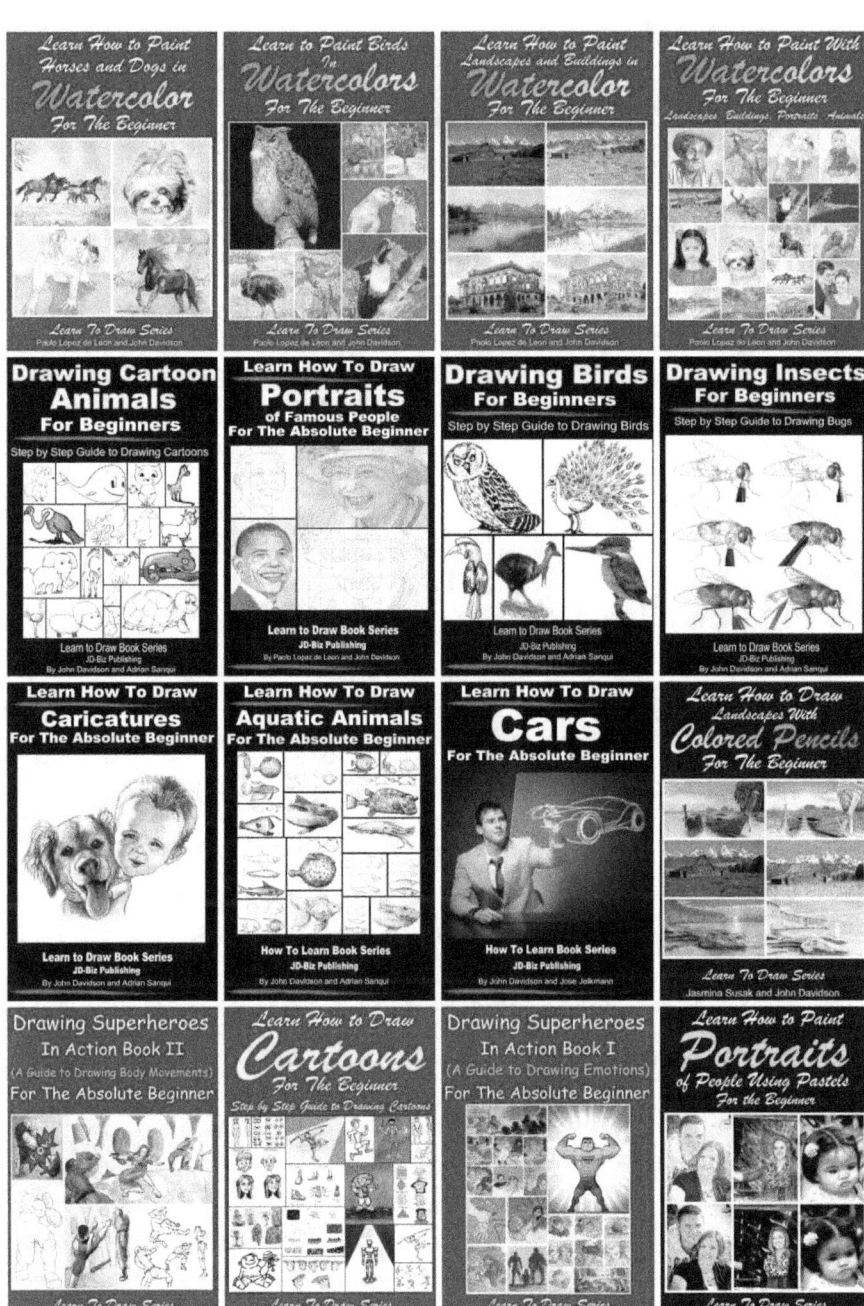

How to Build and Plan Books

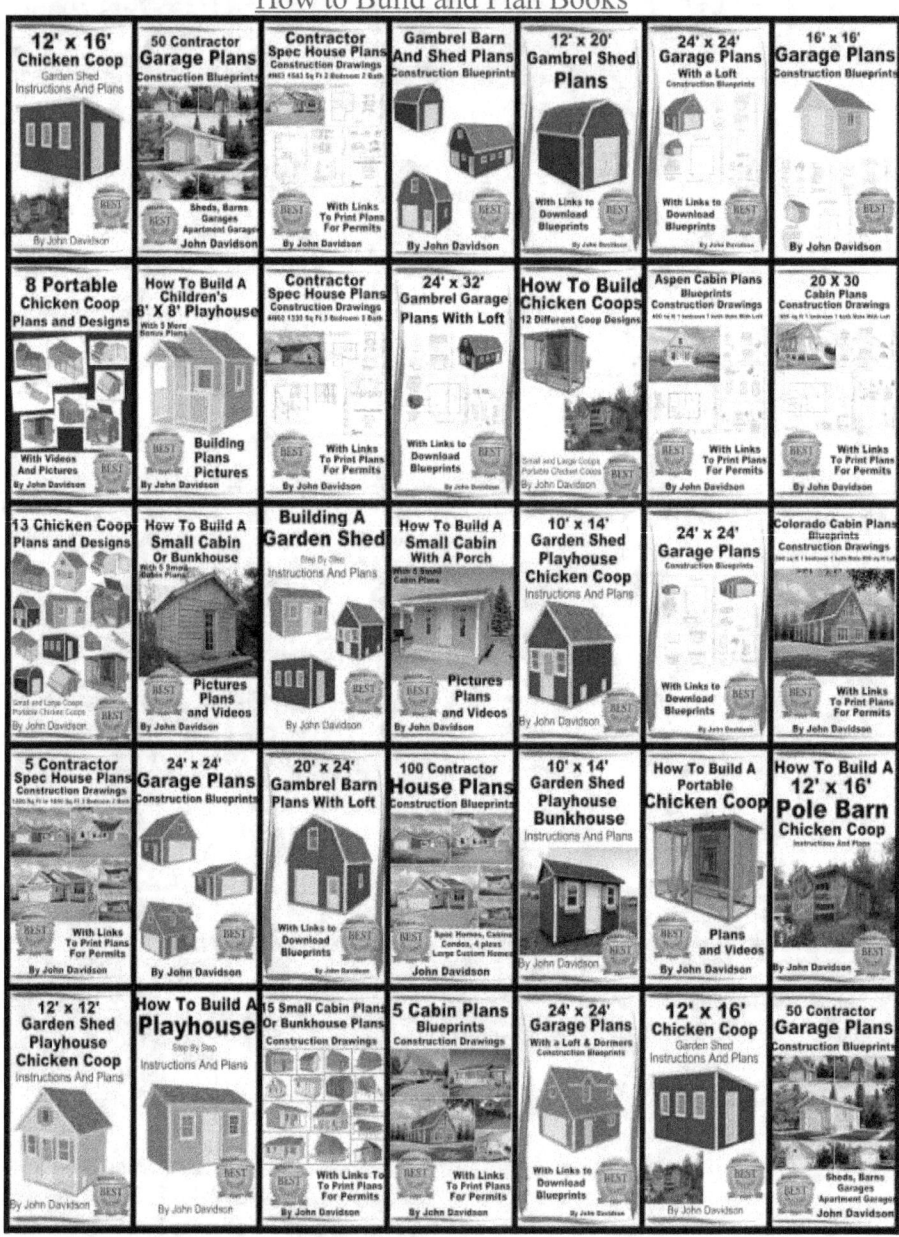

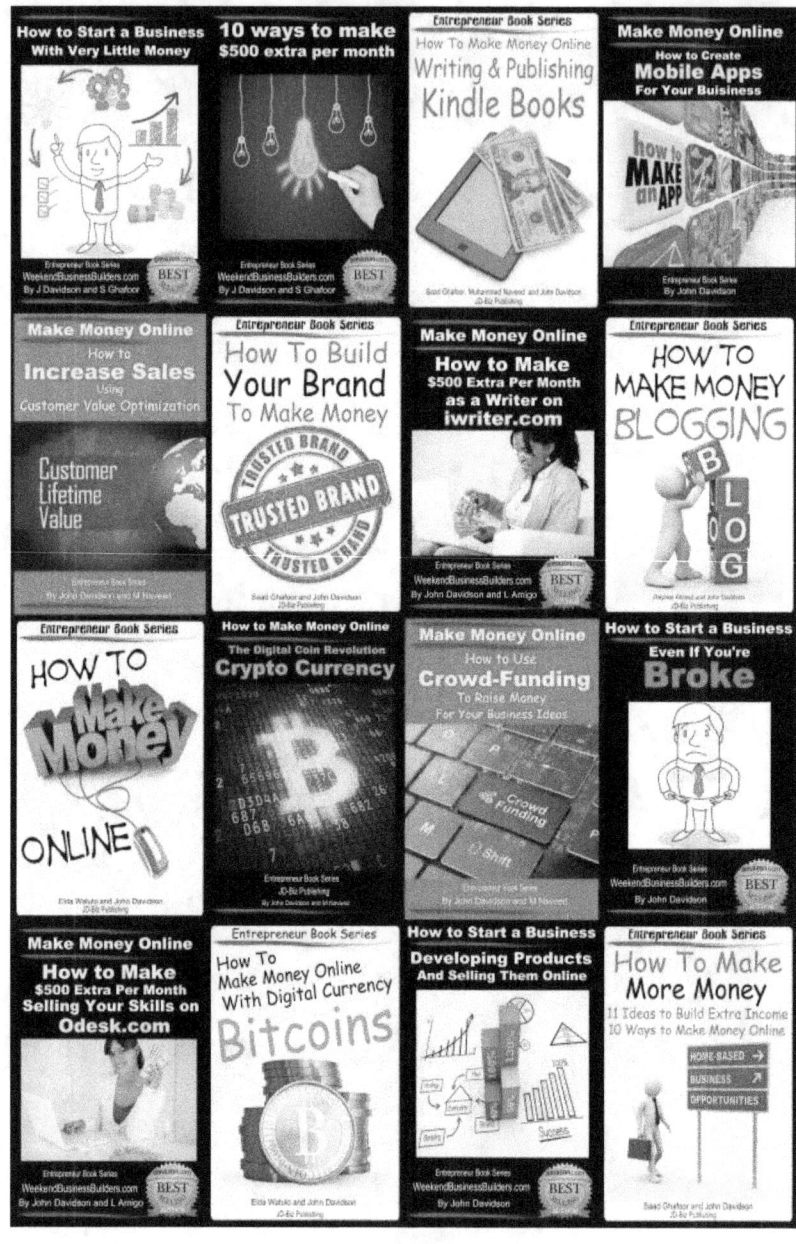

Our books are available at

1. Amazon.com
2. Barnes and Noble
3. Itunes

4. Kobo
5. Smashwords
6. Google Play Books

Publisher

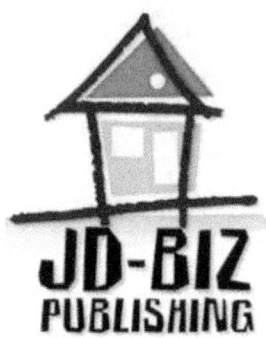

JD-Biz Corp

P O Box 374

Mendon, Utah 84325

http://www.jd-biz.com/

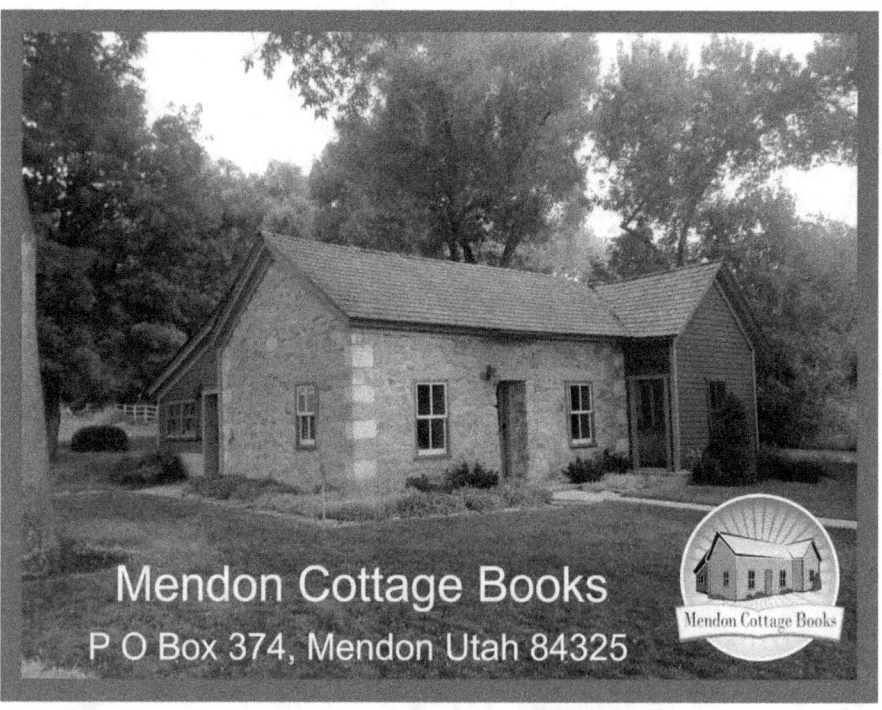

References

http://www.123rf.com/photo_9788798_raw-red-and-white-quinoa-grains-in-jute-sack-on-wood-quinoa-is-grown-in-the-andes-region-and-has-a-h.html?term=quinoa

http://www.123rf.com/photo_20758306_grain-food-selection-in-white-porcelain-dishes-over-hessian-background.html?term=quinoa

http://www.123rf.com/photo_9691361_raw-white-quinoa-grains-in-jute-sack-on-wood-quinoa-is-grown-in-the-andes-and-is-valued-for-its-high.html?term=quinoa

http://www.fotolia.com/id/7367691

http://www.fotolia.com/id/39332640

http://www.fotolia.com/id/40822406

http://www.fotolia.com/id/49549245

http://www.fotolia.com/id/50889876